D1235837

Instructor's Manual For

Nursing Theories and Nursing Practice

Instructor's Manual For

Nursing Theories and Nursing Practice

Shirley Countryman Gordon, PhD, RN
Assistant Professor of Nursing
Florida Atlantic University
College of Nursing
Boca Raton, FL

Cherie Parker, MS, ARNP
West Palm Beach, FL

Reneé Jester, MSN, ARNP
Visiting Assistant Professor of Nursing
Florida Atlantic University
College of Nursing
Boca Raton, FL

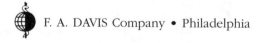
F. A. DAVIS Company • Philadelphia

F. A. Davis Company
1915 Arch Street
Philadelphia, PA 19103
www.fadavis.com

Last digit indicates print number: 10 9 8 7 6 5 4 3 2

Printed in the United States of America

ISBN 0-8036-0605-2

Introduction

The central belief of the book *Nursing Theories and Nursing Practice* is that the study of nursing theory for use in practice, research and education must have roots in the every day practice of nurses. This manual mirrors that belief. Grounding the study of nursing theory in the everyday practice of nursing illuminates the meaning theory has for individual nurses and is essential for closing the gap between theory, research and practice. Closing the gap, allows practitioners and scholars to work together to advance the discipline and professional practice of nursing.

The study of theory for use in nursing practice, education and research requires that students (and faculty) enter a world of unfamiliar terms or terms that are being used in unfamiliar ways (Jacobs-Kramer & Huether, 1988). This unfamiliarity contributes to students seeing theory as mythical, beyond comprehension and having little practical application to the day-to-day world of nursing practice. Introducing students to what theory is, how it is developed, critiqued and analyzed from the perspective of nursing practice demystifies the process of knowledge development (Jacobs-Kramer & Huether, 1988). In other words, it encourages the student to reason on their own about the nature of nursing and to more fully develop their own understanding and appreciation of nursing theory.

The aim of this manual is to facilitate the work of faculty in developing and/or revising courses designed to prepare students to study nursing theory. The manual is intended to be a useful tool in decisions regarding course intent, timing, descriptions, objectives, evaluation and presentation strategies. The study of nursing theory as a continuous, personal journey is reflected throughout the text.

The book and manual are divided into four sections that can be readily used to structure a discrete, undergraduate or graduate course in nursing theory. Sample syllabi using objectives developed for each chapter are provided on pages (to be filled in). (See integration strategies below for ways to reinforce content presented in discrete courses).

Due to limited faculty resources, competing demands for credit hours, economic concerns, student interest, philosophical stances or curriculum design, faculty often choose integrating the study of nursing theory across the curriculum over a discrete theory course (Jacobs-Kramer & Huether, 1988). While such integration is valuable in reinforcing the study of nursing theory over time, there is a risk of fragmenting the content leaving students confused about what theory is and how theory informs practice. The organizational structure (described in Section 4) of the book and manual can be useful in ensuring essential content is not "lost" and that students have a consistent resource guide.

For example, Section 1, Perspectives on Nursing Theory, provides an introduction to nursing theory, guiding questions for the study of nursing theory, as well as a critique and evaluation framework. This section could be used in courses designed to introduce the development of knowledge in nursing or as a content unit in a basic research course.

Instructors designing courses exploring the historical context of nursing will find Section 2, Evolution of Nursing Theory: Essential Influences, a helpful resource. This section presents the theorists who pioneered the development of nursing theory from Nightingale to Patterson and Zderad. Studying the early theorists in this section allows students to trace the footsteps of early theorists and nursing theories used in any part of the curriculum.

Section 3, Nursing Theory in Nursing Practice, Education, Research, Administration, Governance presents the major nursing theories in use at the end of the 20th century with application examples. This content would be useful in guiding students in the context of courses exploring the study of research, education, administration and clinical practice areas.

Section 4, Nursing Theory: Illustrating Processes of Development, presents exemplars of the development of middle-range theory. This content demystifies the process of theory development by providing real life examples of the work of three nurse scholars. Graduate and undergraduate students alike would benefit from reading these stories of scholarship in the process of studying nursing research, nursing theory or courses exploring nursing roles.

Examples of integrating nursing theory are reflected in the sample syllabi located on pages (to be filled in). The syllabi are offered in the hope of supporting creative faculty efforts to integrate the study of nursing theory across the curriculum.

Because time available for course preparation is limited, the manual includes copy ready transparency masters highlighting key points of each chapter. Where possible, the transparencies coincide with the individual chapter objectives and study questions. Faculty wishing to explore strategies for teaching nursing theory are referred to the annotated bibliography provided on pages (to be filled in). Copy ready handouts of study guides for the use of nursing theory in practice, administration and research are also included.

References

Jacobs-Kramer, M.K. & Huether, S.E. (1988). Curricular considerations for teaching nursing theory. *Journal of Professional Nursing*, 4(5), 373-380.

Organization of the Instructor's Manual

This instructor's manual was developed to complement the book Nursing Theories and Nursing Practice by Marilyn Parker. The organizational structure of the manual generally follows the chapters in the text and includes:

Statement of Intent: Provides a brief, broad overview of the intent of individual chapters. The overviews may useful in determining course outlines and reading assignments.

Key Terms: Introduces important terms for each chapter. Instructors may find these useful in constructing test items and in leading classroom discussions.

Chapter Outlines: Expanded chapter outlines provide an opportunity for instructors to quickly review the content and organization of each chapter. The outlines may be useful in organizing lectures and in finding the location of specific chapter content.

Student Objectives/Discussion Questions: Sample objectives/discussion questions have been developed to assist instructors in the process of explicating desired outcomes for the study of nursing theory. The objectives/discussion questions are stated from the learners point of view and incorporate multiple learning levels. Instructors can select those objectives/discussion questions that best meet the learning needs of individual students and reflect overall curricula goals.

Multiple Choice Questions: Multiple choice questions are included for chapters in section one. Answers and page numbers for the questions are provided.

Transparency Masters: Transparency masters are provided to support instructors in lecture preparation and presentation. A list of titles and copy ready transparency masters are located at the end of this manual.

Special Sections: Three special sections are located at the end of the manual. The sections provide sample course syllabi, an annotated bibliography of selected strategies for teaching nursing theory and copy ready study guides for the use of theory in practice, administration and research. These sections are designed to facilitate the development or revision of nursing theory courses.

Contents

SECTION 1
Perspectives on Nursing Theory
Chapter 1
Introduction to Nursing Theory

Statement of Intent: The intent of this chapter is to offer an approach to understanding nursing theory within the context of nursing knowledge, nursing as a discipline, and nursing as a professional practice. Definitions and functions of theory are presented.

Key Terms:

nursing knowledge
discipline
professional practice
theory
paradigms
worldviews
framework

metaparadigm
philosophy
conceptual model
grand theory
middle-range theory
nursing practice theory

Chapter Outline:

Definitions of Nursing Theory
Nursing Theory in the Context of Nursing Knowledge
    Metaparadigm for Nursing
    Nursing Philosophy
    Conceptual Models of Nursing
    Nursing Theories
Types of Nursing Theory
Grand Nursing Theory
    Middle-range Nursing Theory
    Nursing Practice Theory
Nursing's Need for Nursing Theory
    Nursing Is a Discipline
    Expression of Human Imagination
    Domain
    Syntactical and Conceptual Structures
    Specialized Language and Symbols
    Heritage of Literature and Networks of Communication
    Tradition
    Values and Beliefs
    Systems of Education
    Nursing Is a Professional Practice
Nursing Theory and the Future
Summary

Student Objectives/Study Questions:

Following the completion of this chapter students will be able to:

1. Compare and contrast definitions of theory.
2. Describe the usefulness of theory to everyday practice.
3. Identify four phenomena of interest to nursing.
4. Name the primary purpose of nursing theory.
5. List characteristics of nursing as a discipline and a profession.
6. Discuss the importance of conceptualizing nursing as a discipline of knowledge and professional practice.

Multiple-Choice Questions:

1. The purpose of theory is to:
   a.   explain experience
   b.   describe relationships
   c.   project outcomes
   d.   all of the above*
2. The power of theories lies in their ability to:
   a.   Capture the complexity of human nature by the richness of the operational definitions associated with the variables
   b.   Minimize the number of words required to explain phenomena
   c.   Prove that relationships exist among variables studied
   d.   Specify the nature of the relationships that may exist among concepts of interest*
3. The basic building blocks of theories are:
   a.   concepts and their definitions
   b.   statements of relationships
   c.   concepts and statements of relationships*
   d.   empirical indicators
4. Nursing theories:
   a.   are discovered in nature
   b.   serve as exact representations of reality
   c.   are invented by humans*
   d.   cannot be modified
5. A paradigm is defined as a:
   a.   worldview
   b.   general framework
   c.   shared perspectives held by members of a discipline
   d.   all of the above*
6. Science generally evolves as a smooth, regular, continuing path of knowledge development over time.
   a.   True
   b.   False*

*Denotes correct answer.

7. Conceptual levels of knowledge development are influenced by work at other levels.
    a.   True*
    b.   False
8. The dependence of nursing theory development on human imagination is an attribute of nursing as:
    a.   an occupation
    b.   a discipline*
    c.   a vocation
    d.   a profession
9. Theory is always in the process of developing.
    a.   True*
    b.   False
10. The **primary** purpose of nursing theory is to:
    a.   structure nursing knowledge
    b.   demonstrate creativity in nursing
    c.   further development and understanding of nursing practice*
    d.   organize nursing curricula

Transparency Masters (see transparencies 1-1 to 1-6):

1-1   Theories Are Invented
1-2   Theories Are Reflections
1-3   Functions of Theory
1-4   Phenomena of Interest to Nursing
1-5   Characteristics of Nursing as a Discipline
1-6   Characteristics of Nursing as Professional Practice

Chapter 2
Studying Nursing Theory:
Choosing, Analyzing, Evaluating

Statement of Intent: The intent of this chapter is to focus on the study of nursing theory for use in practice, education, administration, research and development. An exercise for the study of nursing theory is provided. Methods of theory analysis and evaluation are discussed.

Key Terms:

studying nursing theory
theory-based practice
values and beliefs
choosing
nursing situation
theory analysis and evaluation
scope

Chapter Outline:

Reasons for Studying Nursing Theory

Questions from Practicing Nurses about Using Nursing Theory
    My Nursing Practice
    My Personal Interests, Abilities, and Experiences
    Resources and Support
    The Theorists, Evidence, and Opinion

Choosing a Nursing Theory to Study

An Exercise for the Study of Nursing Theory
    Enduring Values
    Nursing Situations
    Connecting Values and the Nursing Situation
    Verifying Awareness and Appreciation
    Using Insights to Choose Theory
    Using Authoritative Sources
    Using a Guide to Select a Nursing Theory

Analysis and Evaluation of Nursing Theory
    For Theory Analysis, Consideration Is Given To:
    For Theory Evaluation, Consideration Is Given To:

Summary

Student Objectives/Study Questions:

Following the completion of this chapter students will be able to:

1. Discuss key ways to study nursing theory.
2. Identify and discuss four specific issues important to nurses who consider the study of nursing theory.
3. Describe enduring values and beliefs that guide your nursing practice.
4. Choose a definition of theory that fits a specific purpose for studying nursing theory.
5. Describe the purpose of theory evaluation tools.
6. Discuss important considerations in selecting a theory evaluation guide.

Multiple-Choice Questions:

1. The need to close the gap among theory, research and practice is not considered an urgent issue given the current state of theory development in nursing.
   - a.   True
   - b.   False*
2. To maintain currency in the discipline of nursing all nurses must:
   - a.   be continuing students of nursing
   - b.   join in community to advance nursing knowledge and practice
   - c.   accept obligations to ongoing investigation of nursing theory
   - d.   all of the above*
3. The study and use of nursing theory must have roots in the everyday practice of nursing.
   - a.   True*
   - b.   False
4. Nursing theorists must be removed from practice to maintain objectivity.
   - a.   True
   - b.   False*
5. Ideas and techniques developed through the study of theory and research are:
   - a.   owned by the discipline that developed them
   - b.   claimed for use by individual disciplines*
   - c.   available only to individual researchers
   - d.   useful only to the discipline of nursing
6. Nursing theories considered to be useful must:
   - a.   appear in scholarly nursing journals
   - b.   use specialized language
   - c.   have limited scope
   - d.   be brought into practice*
7. Nursing theorists and nurses in practice:
   - a.   are interested in related but different phenomena
   - b.   do not see nursing in the same context
   - c.   think and work with the same phenomena*
   - d.   require the same knowledge and skills

*Denotes correct answer.

8. Key ways to study nursing include analysis and evaluation.
   a. True*
   b. False
9. The study of nursing theory:
   a. is a simple, short-term endeavor
   b. can be easily undertaken
   c. requires a continuing commitment*
   d. is not essential for expert nursing practice
10. Theories should not be selected for use in practice based on:
   a. congruence with values and beliefs
   b. availability of consultation*
   c. ability to predict nursing phenomena
   d. clarity and simplicity

Transparency Masters (see transparencies 2-1 to 2-5):

2-1   Sensitizing Questions
2-2   Reasons for Studying Nursing Theory
2-3   Central Belief
2-4   Issues Important to the Study of Nursing Theory
2-5   Steps in Choosing a Nursing Theory to Guide Practice

Chapter 3
Guides for Study of Theories for Practice and Administration

Statement of Intent: The intent of this chapter is to offer guidelines for the continuing study of theory for use in nursing practice and administration. Four main questions developed to facilitate the study of nursing theory in practice are presented. Additional questions are offered to facilitate the use of theory in organization and administration of nursing.

Key Terms:

study guide
scope of nursing practice
shared values and beliefs
purpose of nursing
primary sources
theory-based practice
nursing practice
nursing administration

Chapter Outline:

Study of Theory for Nursing Practice

A Guide for Study of Nursing Theory for Use in Practice

Study of Theory for Nursing Administration

Summary

Student Objectives/Study Questions:

Following the completion of this chapter students will be able to:

1. Discuss the importance of identifying values and beliefs shared by groups of nurses.
2. Identify concepts of interest in studying nursing theory for use in practice.
3. Identify concepts of interest in studying nursing theory for use in nursing administration.
4. Demonstrate the use of study guides to direct the analysis and evaluation of selected nursing theorists.

Multiple Choice Questions:

1. The scope of nursing practice is limited.
   - a.   True
   - b.   False*
2. Nurses working together as colleagues often realize that:
   - a.   their views of nursing are not compatible
   - b.   they share the same values and beliefs*
   - c.   the study of nursing theory does not enhance their work
   - d.   none of the above
3. Responses to guiding questions about theory in practice can be found in the following resources:
   - a.   nursing literature
   - b.   audiovisual materials
   - c.   electronic resources
   - d.   all of the above*
4. Study of the use of theory in nursing practice should be undertaken by:
   - a.   nursing students at all levels
   - b.   practicing nurses and students*
   - c.   advanced practice nurses
   - d.   practicing staff nurses
5. Nursing theory can be used to guide nursing practice, administration, and research.
   - a.   True*
   - b.   False

Transparency Masters (see Transparencies 3-1 and 3-2):

3-1   Study of Nursing Theory for Use in Practice Guide
3-2   Study of Nursing Theory for Use in Nursing Administration Guide

*Denotes correct answer.

SECTION 2
Evolution of Nursing Theory: Essential Influences

Chapter 4
Florence Nightingale
Caring Actualized: A Legacy for Nursing

Statement of Intent: This chapter explores the life of Florence Nightingale and her contributions to nursing. A biographical account is presented covering her education, travel, spiritual background and Crimean War experiences. The medical environment of the 1800s and her views of women during that time are also presented. An overview is provided for the foundations of Nightingale's model of nursing and how it is interpreted today.

Key Terms:

spirituality
Crimean War
moral authority
atmosphere
environment
sickness
ontagionism
feminism
expressions of caring
laws of nursing
laws of health
health of houses

observation
personal cleanliness
petty management
light
cleanliness of rooms
ventilation and warming
bed and bedding
taking food
what food?
noise
chattering hopes and advices
variety

Chapter Outline:

Introducing the Theorist
Early Life and Education: The Seeds of Caring Planted
Spirituality: The Roots of Nightingale's Caring
War: Caring Actualized
The Medical Milieu
The Feminist Context of Nightingale's Caring
Ideas about Nursing: Expressions of Caring
Nightingale's Assumptions
Summary

Student Objectives/Study Questions:

Following the completion of this chapter students will be able to:

1. Summarize significant events in Nightingale's life that led her to nursing and influenced her model of nursing.
2. Compare and contrast the medical milieu of the 1800s with the medical milieu of today.
3. Discuss Nightingale's feminist view.
4. Analyze expressions of caring from Nightingale's theory.
5. Discuss Nightingale's assumptions and how they are useful in nursing today.
6. Understand Nightingale's conception of nursing.
7. Apply Nightingale's Environmental Model to the practice of nursing.
8. Identify and discuss the four major factors that influenced Nightengale's model of nursing.

Transparency Masters (see transparencies 4-1 to 4-3):

4-1   Health of Houses
4-2   Major Factors Influencing Nightingale's Model
4-3   Nightingale's Assumptions

Chapter 5
Hildegard E. Peplau
The Process of Practice-based Theory Development

Statement of Intent: The purpose of this chapter is to familiarize the reader with Hildegard Peplau as person, teacher, pioneer in psychiatric nursing and theorist. The completion of the chapter discusses how Peplau's theory has impacted students, theory development and how it springs from practice.

Key Terms:

nurse-patient relationship
subject
decoding
categorizing
transcribing
participant observer
spectator observer
random observation

Chapter Outline:

Introducing the Theorist

The Experience of a Third Generation Peplau Student

Peplau's Process of Practice-Based Theory Development

Peplau's Practice-based Process and a Program of Research
    Follow-up Study
    Negative Thinking
    Testing an Intervention
    Testing the Intervention with At-Risk Women

Peplau for the Future

Summary

Student Objectives/Study questions:

Following the completion of this chapter students will be able to:

1. Discuss the history and accomplishments of Hildegard Peplau.
2. Discuss the process of practice-based theory development as described by Peplau

3. Explain the natural progression from inductive to deductive research within the process of practice-based theory development.
4. Understand the importance of practice-based theory development and usage.

Transparency Masters (see transparencies 5-1 to 5-3):

5-1   Life History
5-2   3-step Process of Practice-Based Theory Development
5-3   Induction to Deduction

Chapter 6
Ernestine Wiedenbach
Wiedenbach's Clinical Nursing:
A Helping Art

Statement of Intent: The intent of this chapter is to review the theoretical work of Ernestine Wiedenbach.

Key Terms:

prescription
prescriptive theory
philosophy
integration of body, mind and spirit
motivating factors
realities
nursing's central purpose
deliberate action
agent
recipient
framework
goal
means

Chapter Outline:

Introducing the Theorist
The Evolution of Wiedenbach's Prescriptive Theory
The Prescriptive Theory
Wiedenbach's Theory and Clinical Practice
Wiedenbach's Theory and Clinical Teaching
Summary

Student Objectives/Study Questions:

Following the completion of this chapter students will be able to:

1. Describe the essentials of prescriptive theory.
2. List the essence of a philosophy according to Wiedenbach.
3. Discuss features of the realities of nursing practice.

4. List four responsibilities of the nurse as agent.
5. Identify five features of practice realities.
6. Choose a nursing situation and describe it using Wiedenbach's realities of practice.

Transparency Masters (see transparencies 6-1 to 6-7):

6-1   Essence of a Philosophy
6-2   Prescriptions Specify
6-3   Kinds of Deliberate Action
6-4   Essential Ingredients of Prescriptive Theory
6-5   Features of Practice Realities
6-6   Steps in Reaching Goals
6-7   Theory and Clinical Practice

Chapter 7
Dorothy Johnson
Behavioral Systems Model for Nursing

Statement of Intent: The intent of this chapter is to provide an overview of Dorothy Johnson's behavioral systems model for nursing. This chapter also provides an overview of the use of the model in nursing practice, administration, research and education.

Key Terms:

paradigmatic origins
systems theorists
behavioral systems model
wholeness and order
stabilization
reorganization
hierarchic interaction
dialectical contradiction
general systems
plasticity
subsystem
homeorhesis
homeostasis
external regulator
motivational choice

developmental theory
pragmatic origins
achievement subsystem
affiliative subsystem
aggressive/protective subsystem
dependency subsystem
eliminative subsystem
ingestive subsystem
restorative subsystem
sexual subsystem
person
environment
health
nursing and nursing therapeutics

Chapter Outline:

Role of the Model in Nursing Practice, Administration, Research, and Education
    Research
    Education
    Nursing Practice and Administration
Summary

Student Objectives/Study Questions

Following the completion of this chapter students will be able to:

1. Discuss paradigmatic origins of Johnson's model.
2. Discuss the five core principles of Dorothy Johnson's behavioral systems model.
3. Identify the eight subsystems of Dorothy Johnson's behavioral systems model and discuss their interrelationship.
4. Describe Johnson's definition of person, environment, health and nursing.
5. Discuss the role of the behavioral systems model in nursing practice, administration, research and education.

Transparency Masters (see transparencies 7-1 to 7-4):

7-1   Paradigmatic Origins
7-2   Five Core Principles
7-3   Subsystems
7-4   Definitions

Chapter 8
Myra Levine
Conservation Model: A Model for the Future

Statement of Intent: This chapter explores the demographics and educational background of Myra Levine, explains the assumptions and values of her nursing theory and demonstrates how this theory could be useful in practice.

Key Terms

conservation
adaptation
wholeness
redundancy
specificity
organismic
environmental fit
trophicognosis
internal and external environment
single integrity
structure

Chapter Outline

Introducing the Theorist

Introduction to the Foundations of Clinical Nursing

The Conservation Model Informed by the Adjunctive Sciences

The Composition of the Conservation Model

Philosophical Notes
    Assumptions
    Values

The Model's Fit with Practice
    Use of the Conservation Model in Practice
    The Conservation Model as a Model for Community-based Care—
        A Modification of the Model

Research Based on the Conservation Model

The Conservation Model in the Twenty-first Century

Summary

Student Objectives/Study Questions

Following the completion of this chapter students will be able to:

1. Recall the education and historical contributions of Levine's theory development.
2. Identify the basic values and assumptions of the conservation model.
3. Discuss how the conservation model can be applied to a variety of practice settings.
4. Explain how the conservation model impacts the nursing process.

Transparency Masters (see transparencies 8-1 to 8-3):

8-1 Assumptions
8-2 Values
8-3 Organismic Responses

Chapter 9
Ida Jean Orlando (Pelletier)
The Dynamic Nurse-Patient Relationship

Statement of Intent: This chapter reviews the theory of dynamic nurse-patient relationships. This segment offers an opportunity to come to know Ida Orlando, author of the theory, and to explore potential applications of her theory to current nursing practice and research.

Key Terms:

nonlinear nursing process
client or person
needs
perceptions
thoughts
feelings of nurse
deliberative action
symbolic environment

Chapter Outline:

Introducing the Theorist

A Conversation with the Theorist

Assumptions of the Theory

Major Theoretical Concepts

Relevance of the Theory for Nursing Practice
    Goals
    Fit
    Understandability
    Sufficiently General
    Control

Applicability in Today's Health-Care System

Summary

Student Objectives/Study Questions

Following the completion of the chapter students will be able to:

1. Review the demographic and historical background of Ida Orlando, nurse theorist.
2. Be able to articulate the goals, fit, understandability and generalizability of the dynamic nurse-patient relationship.
3. Select the strengths and weaknesses of the Orlando nursing theory.

Transparency Masters (see transparencies 9-1 and 9-2):

9-1   Quote from Orlando
9-2   Goals: fit, understandibility, generalizability, control

Chapter 10
Lydia Hall
The Care, Core, and Cure Model

Statement of Intent: This chapter represents the story of Lydia Hall and the development of the Loeb Center for Nursing and Rehabilitation. An overview of Hall's care, core and cure model and its implications for nursing practice and research is provided.

Key Terms:

Loeb Center for Nursing and
    Rehabilitation
care
core
cure
circles
biological crisis
acute crisis
nurturing

direct care
person
body
disease
intimate bodily care
nurturer
comforter
therapeutic use of self

Chapter Outline:

Introducing the Theorist

Historical Background

Vision of Nursing

Care, Core, and Cure
    Care
    Core
    Cure

The Loeb Center for Nursing and Rehabilitation

Implications for Nursing Practice

Implications for Nursing Research

Summary

Student Objectives/Study Questions:

Following the completion of this chapter students will be able to:

1. Discuss Lydia Hall's vision of nursing.
2. Define care, cure and core as it applies to Hall's model.

3. Illustrate the care, core and cure model and discuss how the circles change in relationship to patient progress.
4. Discuss the philosophy of the Loeb Center and nursing care that was provided.
5. Understand implications for practice and research.
6. Discuss the future of the care, core and cure model.

Transparency Masters (see transparencies 10-1 to 10-3):

10-1   Aspects of Person as Patient
10-2   Loeb Center RNs
10-3   Deterrents to Replicating the Loeb Center Model

Chapter 11
Virginia Avenel Henderson
(1897-1996)

Statement of Intent: The intent of this chapter is to introduce Virginia Henderson's definition of nursing and 14 basic care components. The chapter also provides an overview of Henderson's work in the areas of international nursing, nursing education and highlights her career in library research and development.

Key Terms:

nature of nursing
unique function
independent practitioner
care components
basic nursing care
fundamental needs
nursing and non-nursing functions
plan of care
understanding of self
art of nursing
evaluating quality of care
nursing studies index

Chapter Outline:

Introducing the Theorist

Personal Background

The Search for a Personal Definition of Nursing

Influence on International Nursing

IInfluence on Nursing Education

Influence on Practice

Influence on Library Research and Development

Summary

Student Objectives/Study Questions

Following the completion of this chapter students will be able to:

1. Describe the significance of Virginia Henderson's definition of nursing.
2. Discuss Henderson's rationale for legitimate nursing activities.

3. Identify components that encompass basic nursing care.
4. Describe Henderson's view of sequencing learning activities.
5. Identify three questions Henderson used to evaluate patients' perceptions of quality care.

Transparency Masters (see transparencies 11-1 to 11-7):

11-1 People Influencing Henderson's Search for a Personal Definition of Nursing
11-2 Questions Directing Henderson's Search for a Definition of Nursing
11-3 Henderson's Definition of Nursing
11-4 Henderson's 14 Basic Care Components
11-5 Henderson's Basic Nursing Care Components
11-6 Questions Henderson Used to Evaluate Nursing Care
11-7 Statement on Independent Practice

Chapter 12
Patterson and Zderad
Humanistic Nursing Theory with Clinical Applications*

Statement of Intent: This chapter provides an overview of Humanistic Nursing theory developed by Patterson and Zderad. The philosophical and methodological background is explored. Uses of the theory in nursing practice, clinical supervision and research are presented.

Key Terms:

humanistic nursing
existentialism
lived experience
call
response
in-between
phenomenological inquiry
nursing situation
receptivity
reflective immersion
humanizing experience
well-being

more being
being and becoming
nurturing
choosing
gestalt
"all at once"
being with
doing with
transactional
shared human experience
"knowing place"

Chapter Outline:

---

*This chapter in the student edition was reprinted with permission of the National League for Nursing, New York

Clinical Applications of Humanistic Nursing Theory
    Nurse's Reflection on Nursing
    Patient's Reflection on Nursing
    Uses of the Theory in Clinical Supervision
Use of the Theory in Research
Developing a Community of Nurses
The Call of Humanity

Student objectives/Study Questions:

Following the completion of this chapter students will be able to:
1. Identify the phases of the humanistic nursing theory.
2. Define nursing from the perspective of humanistic nursing.
3. Discuss humanistic nursing.
4. Describe a nursing situation from the perspective of humanistic nursing.
5. Identify and describe Patterson and Zderad's 11 phenomena of nursing.

Transparency Masters (see transparencies 12-1 to 12-6):

12-1   World of Others and Things
12-2   Shared Human Experience
12-3   Patient and Nurse Gestalts "between"
12-4   Phases of Humanistic Nursing Inquiry
12-5   Nurse Complimentarily Synthesizing Others
12-6   Eleven Phenomenon of Nursing

SECTION 3
Nursing Theory in Nursery Practice, Education, Research, Administration, Governance
Chapter 13
Dorothea E. Orem
The Self-Care Deficit Nursing Theory

Statement of Intent: The intent of this chapter is to provide an overview of Orem's self care deficit theory of nursing and its direction for advancing nursing science and professional practice. The chapter also provides views of human beings specific to nursing by Dorothea Orem.

Key Terms:

self-care
self-care deficit
general theory
nursing systems
self-care agency
therapeutic self-care demand
nursing agency
self-care requisites
wholly compensatory
partly compensatory
supportive-educative nursing systems
social utility
basic conditioning factors
self-care agency scale

Chapter Outline:

Part 1

Introducing the Theorist

Views of Human Beings Specific to Nursing
    Nursing-specific Views
    Broader Views
    Model Building and Theory Development
    Conclusion

Part 2 Self-Care Deficit Theory of Nursing: Directions for Advancing Nursing Science and Professional Practice

Orem's General Theory of Nursing

The Development of Nursing Science

The Cross-cultural and International Scope of Research

Uses of Orem's Theory in Nursing Practice: An Overview

Summary

Student Objectives/Discussion Questions

Following the completion of this chapter students will be able to:

1. Explain the concept of self-care.
2. Discuss Orem's view of the role of nursing.
3. Understand the concepts of the self-care deficit theory.
4. Define wholly compensatory, partly compensatory, and supportive educative system.
5. Discuss the use of the self-care deficit theory in nursing and its use in research.

Transparency Masters (see transparencies 13-1 to 13-3):

13-1   Sensitizing Question
13-2   Role of Nursing
13-3   Self-Care Deficit Theory of Nursing Concepts

Chapter 14
Martha E. Rogers
Rogers' Science of
Unitary Human Beings

Statement of Intent: This chapter introduces Martha Rogers: person, scholar, nurse, and theorist. The Science of Unitary Human Beings theory is introduced and explained. Finally exploration of the uses of Rogers's nursing theory in practice, research and future implications are reviewed.

Key Terms:

openness

nonlinear domain

resonancy

integrality

unitary humans beings

patterning

helicy

homeostasis

pandimensional view

homo spatialis

homo sapiens

mutual process

dynamic equilibrium

innovative growing diversity

energy fields

irreducible human beings

Chapter Outline:

Part 1: Science of Unitary Human Being

Introducing the Theorist

The Science of Unitary Human Beings: Overview
    Rogers's Worldview
    Postulates of Rogerian Nursing Science
    Principles of Homeodynamics

Theories Identified by Rogers
    Barrett's Theory of Power as Knowing Participation in Change

Examples of Proposed Theories Being Developed by Other Rogerian Scholars
    Theory of Perceived Dissonance
    The Theory of Sentience Evolution
    Theory of Healthiness
    Enfolding Health-as-Wholeness-and-HarmonyRogerian Science-based Practice
    and Research
    Practice
    Research

Part 2: Nursing Science in the New Millennium: Practice and Research Within Roger's Science of Unitary Human Beings

Rogerian Practice Models
    Barrett's Rogerian Practice Methodology for Health Patterning
    Cowling's Pattern Appreciation Practice Method
    Toward a Synthesis of Rogerian Practice Models
    Pattern Maanifestation Knowing and Appreciation
    Voluntary Mutual Patterning
    Selected Midrange Rogerian Practice Theories
    Theory of Power as Knowing Participation in Change
    Theory of Perceived Dissonance
    Theory of Kaleidoscoping in Life's Turbulence
    Enfolding Health-as-Wholeness-Harmony
    Personalized Nursing LIGHT Practice Model

Research Within the Science of Unitary Human Beings
    Methodological Issues
    Criteria for Rogerian Inquiry
    Potential Rogerian Research Designs
    Selecting a Focus of Rogerian Inquiry
    Measurement of the Concept
    Rogerian Process of Inquiry
    The Unitary Field Pattern Portrait Research Method
    Unitary Case Inquiry

Summary

Student Objectives/Study Questions:

Following the completion of this chapter students will be able to:

1. Recall the historical, educational and personal information relevant to Martha Rogers's life as a nurse theorist.
2. Categorize and define the unusual terms used in the Science of Unitary Human Beings nursing theory.
3. Discuss how to operationalize the Rogerian theory in practice and research.
4. Identify research questions that would work well with the Rogers's nursing theory.
5. Compare and contrast homeodynamics with homeostasis.

Transparency Masters (see transparencies 14-1 to 14-4):

14-1   Historical Perspective of Martha Rogers
14-2   Rogers's Unique View of Nursing
14-3   Rogers's Principles of Homeodynamics
14-4   Rogerian Practice Model

Chapter 15
Rosemarie Parse
The Human Becoming School of Thought: A Guide for Research and Practice

Statement of Intent: This chapter reviews the theoretical work of Rosemarie Parse and examines the various ways the Human Becoming school of thought can be applied to nursing practice and research.

Key Terms:

human becoming
true presence
discipline
profession
totality paradigm
meaning
imaging
valuing
languaging
revealing-concealing

enabling-limiting
connecting-separating
powering
rhythmicity
transcendence
simultaneity paradigm
paradoxes
unitary humans
all-at-onceness

Chapter Outline:

Research on Human Becoming
    Parse's Phenomenological Method
    Hermeneutic Method and Evaluation Method

Nursing Leadership from a Human Becoming Perspective: One Leader's Story
    Processes of Leading in Change
    The First 5 Years
    Challenges of Change

A Nursing Regulatory Decisioning Model

The Human Becoming Theory in Teaching-Learning

Student Objectives/Study Questions:

Following the completion of this chapter students will be able to:

1. Define the discipline and profession of nursing as implicated by Rosemarie Parse.
2. Critique the reasons for changing man-living-health to human becoming decision made by Parse.
3. Identify the nine assumptions underlying the three major themes of Parse's human becoming theory.
4. Define and discuss Parse's hermanuetic research method.

Transparency Masters (see transparencies 15-1 to 15-4):

15-1   Discipline and Profession
15-2   Transition from Man-Living-health to human becoming
15-3   Assumptions-themes
15-4   Research methodologies

Chapter 16
Margaret A. Newman
Health as Expanding Consciousness

Statement of Intent: The intent of this chapter is to provide an overview of Margaret Newman's theory of health as expanding conciousness. This chapter also provides an in-depth look at this use of the theory in the research process.

Key Terms:

health as expanding consciousness
unitary energy fields
unitary being perspective
caring in the human health experience
particulate-deterministic paradigm
interactive-integrative perspective
unitary-transformative perspective
person-environment interaction
choice point
potential freedom
binding
unbinding
entering
choice

decentering
real freedom
being
doing
mutual transformation
hermeneutic dialectic-hermeneutic
HEC research process
interview
transcription
narrative
diagram
follow-up
research as praxis

Chapter Outline:

Introducing the Theorist: The Unfolding of Margaret Newman's Theory of Health as Expanding Consciousness

The Debut of Margaret Newman's Theory

Uniqueness and Wholeness of Pattern

A New Paradigm Emerges

Sequential Configurations of Pattern Evolving Over Time

Insights Occurring as Choice Points of Action Potential

Health as Expanding Consciousness

The Mutuality of the Nurse–Client Interaction in the Process of Pattern Recognition

Hermeneutic Dialectic Method of Research

The Health as Expanding Consciousness Research Process

Theory as Moving Intuition and Evolving Insights

Student Objectives/Study Questions

Following the completion of this chapter students will be able to:

1. Understand Newman's definition of consciousness.
2. Discuss the distinct paradigmatic views of caring in the human health experience.
3. Explain the seven stages of binding and unbinding.
4. Describe mutual transformation in the nurse client interaction.
5. Understand the HEC research process.

Transparency Masters (see transparencies 16-1 to 16-3):

16-1   Stages of Binding and Unbinding

16-2   Caring in the Human Health Experience

16-3   HEC Research Process

Chapter 17
Imogene M. King
Theory of Goal Attainment

Statement of Intent: The intent of this chapter is to explore the evolution of King's theory and describe the state of the art in terms of the work being done in relation to the application of King's conceptual framework and theory in a variety of areas: practice, administration, education and research.

Key Terms:

system

nation

action

interaction

goal setting

transaction

outcome

interpersonal system

goal attainment

nonclinical nursing situation

empathy

health of a social system

health of systems

space

perceptual awareness

standardized nursing language

Chapter Outline:

Part 1: Theory of Goal Attainment

Introducing the Theorist

Worldview: King's Conceptual System and Middle-Range Theory of Goal Attainment

Initial Ideas: The Beginning

Philosophy of Science

Design of a Conceptual System
    Process for Developing a Concept
    King's Conceptual System

King's Theory of Goal Attainment
    Transaction Process Model
    Documentation System
    Goal Attainment Scale
    Use of King's Conceptual System and Theory
    Nursing Education
    Practice
    Family Health
    Community Health
    Use in Hospitals

Student Objectives/Study Questions:

Following the completion of this chapter students will be able to:

1. Explore the evolution of King's theory from her personal writings.
2. Classify and discuss a variety of literature related to King's theory.
3. Identify appropriate research questions for implementation of King's theory in research.
4. Compare and contrast medical and nursing research techniques according to King.
5. Discuss outcome-based research and identify examples from cited literature.

Transparency Masters (see transparencies 17-1 to 17-5):

17-1   King's Conceptual System
17-2   Definition of System
17-3   Process of Concept Development and Validation
17-4   Sensitizing Question
17-5   Goal of Nursing

Chapter 18
Sister Callista Roy
The Roy Adaptation Model

Statement of Intent: The intent of this chapter is to describe the use of the Roy adaptation model for developing knowledge. Research directed by the model is summarized. The chapter presents a research exemplar with hearing-impaired elderly.

Key Terms:

humanism
veritivity
cosmic unity
general systems theory
holistic adaptive system
coping processes
adaptation
adaptation level
adaptive modes
internal environment
external environment
transform
cognator-regulator
stabilizer-innovator
cognitive adaptation processing
self-consistency
clinical science of nursing

Chapter Outline:

Application of the Model (Research Exemplar): Elderly Patients with Hearing
    Impairment
    Study Design
    Research Hypothesis
    Sample
    Major Variables
    Data Collection
    Findings
Nursing Practice Implications of the Research

Application of Exemplar

Summary

Student Objectives/Study Questions:

Following the completion of this chapter students will be able to:

1. Identify four categories for assessing behavior using the Roy adaptation model.
2. Describe topics for research guided by the Roy adaptation model.
3. Discuss Roy's view of the clinical science of nursing.
4. Explain the applicability of cognitive adaptation processing and self-consistency to a specific nursing situation.
5. Appreciate the development of a research program.

Transparency Masters (see transparencies 18-1 to 18-4):

18-1   Adaptive Modes
18-2   Central Belief of the Roy adaptation model
18-3   Topics for Research
18-4   Knowledge Development Strategies Based on the Roy adaptation model

Chapter 19
Betty Neuman
Neuman Systems Model and
Global Applications

Statement of Intent: The intent of this chapter is to explain the Neuman systems model, share global applications of the model and provide a bibiliography to facilitate further study.

Key Terms:

client
system
complete whole
interrelationship
negentrophy
wellness state
entrophy
stressors
lines of resistance
lines of defense
basic structure

Chapter Outline:

Introducing the Theorist

The Neuman Systems Model
    Propositions
    The Conceptual Model
    Client-Client System
    Flexible Line of Defense
    Normal Line of Defense
    Lines of Resistance
    Basic Structure
    Five Client Variables
    Environment
    Health
    Nursing
    Prevention as Intervention
    Nursing Tools for Model Implementation

Student Objectives/Study Questions:

Following the completion of this chapter students will be able to:

1. Identify and differentiate among primary, secondary and tertiary prevention as discussed in Neuman's theory.
2. Define and discuss Neuman's five client variables.

Transparency Masters (see transparencies 19-1 to 19-3):

19-1   Betty Neuman's Systems Model
19-2   Neuman's Five Client Variables
19-3   Role of Nurse

Chapter 20
Jean Watson
Theory of Human Caring

Statement of Intent: The intent of this chapter is to provide an overview of the major conceptual elements of the original theory of human caring and its evolution. Watson provides a translation of the original carative factors into clinical caritas processes. A practice demonstration is provided to demonstrate the philosophy and science of human caring in a nurse-directed facility.

Key Terms:

carative factors
curative factors
transpersonal caring relationship
caring moment/caring occasion
expanded view of self and person
caring-healing consciousness
phenomenal field/unitary consciousness
caring-healing modalities
clinical caratis
caritas processes
transpersonal caring theory
core of nursing
"trim"
health/healing
Denver Nursing Project
caring leadership

Chapter Outline:

Part 1

Introducing the Theorist

Theory of Human Caring

Overview of the Theory

Original and Evolving 10 Carative Factors
    Clinical Caritas and Caritas Processes
    Original Carative Factors
    From Carative Factors to Clinical Caritas Processes

Transpersonal Caring Relationship
  Assumptions of Transpersonal Caring Relationship
Caring Moment/Caring Occasion
Caring (Healing) Consciousness
Implications of the Caring Model
Summary

Part 2: Caring for the Human Spirit in the Workplace
The Human Being, The Human Spirit, and Human Relationships
Health/Healing
The Denver Nursing Project in Human Caring (The Caring Center)
Caring Theory in New Contexts
Summary

Student Objectives/Study Questions:

Following the completion of this chapter students will be able to:

1. Understand the original carative factors and compare to clinical caritas processes.
2. Discuss the evolution of the original ten carative factors into clinical caritas process.
3. Define transpersonal caring relationships and discuss assumptions of transpersonal relationships.
4. Understand caring moment/caring occasion and caring consciousness.
5. Discuss implications of the caring model.
6. Examine the human care theory in leadership for an organization, business or work group.

Transparency Masters (see transparencies 20-1 to 20-5):

20-1   Major Conceptual Themes
20-2   Original Carative Factors 1-5
20-3   Original Carative Factors 6-10
20-4   Role of Consciousness
20-5   Effective Caring Leader Questions

Chapter 21
Madeleine M. Leininger
Theory of Culture Care Diversity and Universality

Statement of Intent: The intent of this chapter is to provide an overview of the theory of culture care diversity and universality. The purpose, goal, assumptions, theoretical hunches and general features of the theory are presented. Explanation of the sunrise model and definition of theory terms are addressed.

Key Terms:

transcultural

transcultural nursing

culture care

anthropology

caring

holistic knowledge

holistic health

generic care

local or folk care

kinship and social factors

religious and philosophical factors

political and legal factors

cultural values and lifeways

technological factors

educational factors

economic factors

environmental context

influences

care expression patterns and practices

culturally congruent care

domain of inquiry

Chapter Outline:

Part 1

Introducing the Theorist

Culture Care Diversity and Unversality: A Worldwide Nursing Theory

Factors Leading to the Theory

Rationale for Transcultural Nursing: Signs and Need

Major Theoretical Tenets
> Theoretical Assumptions: Purpose, Goal, and Definitions of the Theory
> Assumptins of the Theory
> Orientational Theory Definitions

Sunrise Model: A Conceptual Guide to Knowledge Discovery
Current Status of the Theory

Future of the Culture Care Theory

Summary

Part 2: The Ethnonursing Research Method

The Ethnonursing Research Method
    Qualitative Paradigm and Quantitive Paradigm
    Purpose and Philosophical Features
    Domain of Inquiry
    Key and General Informants
    Enablers
    Qualitative Criteria to Evaluate Ethnonursing Studies
    Four Phases of Ethnonursing Analysis for Qualitative Data
    The Steps in the Ethnonursing Research Process

Culture Care Theory and Nursing Practice
    The Three Care Modes and the Sunrise Model
    The Use of Culture Care Research Findings
    Culture Care of Lebanese Muslims in the United States
    Culture Care of Elderly Anglo- and African Americans
    Culture Care of Mexican-American Pregnant Women

Summary

Student Objectives/ Study Questions:

Following the completion of this chapter students will be able to:

1. Discuss the rationale for transcultural nursing.
2. Define transcultural nursing.
3. Identify and discuss the purpose and goal of the culture care theory.
4. Discuss the major theoretical tenets of the theory.
5. Examine the current status of the theory and its future direction.
6. Discuss culture care research and its importance to practice.

Transparency Masters (see transparencies 21-1 to 21-5):

21-1   Rationale for Transcultural Nursing
21-2   Transcultural Nursing
21-3   Culturally Congruent Care Modalities
21-4   Purpose of Cultural Care Theory
21-5   Goal of Cultural Care Theory

Chapter 22
Anne Boykin and
Savina O. Schoenhofer
Nursing as Caring

Statement of Intent: The intent of this chapter is to provide an overview of the theory of nursing as caring. Assumptions and key terms are identified. Answers are provided to the most frequently asked questions regarding the theory. Nursing as caring is explored in various nursing roles with a lived experience presented in the advanced practice setting.

Key Terms:

caring
focus and intention of caring
nursing situation
personhood
call for nursing
nursing response
caring between
lived meaning of nursing as caring
patterns of knowing
    personal
    empirical
    ethical
    aesthetic

authentic presence
humanness
coming to know self
caring in the moment
person-with-person caring
caring person
calls for nursing

Chapter Outline:

Part 1

Introducing the Theorists
    Anne Boykin
    Savina O. Schoenhofer

Nursing as Caring: An Overview of a General Theory of Nursing
    Assumptions
    Caring
    Key Themes
    Focus and Intention of Nursing
    Nursing Situation
    Personhood
    Call for Nursing

Student Objectives/Study Questions:

Following the completion of this chapter students will be able to:

1. Discuss the meaning of caring, the assumptions and the key themes of nursing as caring.
2. Understand how coming to know self as caring is facilitated.
3. Compare/contrast nursing as caring with the nursing process
4. Explore the use of nursing as caring in a nursing situation.
5. Appreciate the use of nursing as caring in the different roles of nursing.
6. Present or share a nursing situation in the form of a case presentation, story, poem, or any other art form.

Transparency Masters (see transparencies 22-1 to 22-5):

22-1   Assumptions
22-2   Caring
22-3   Key Themes
22-4   Coming to Know Self
22-5   Frequently Asked Questions

SECTION 4
Nursing Theory: Illustrating Processes of Development

Chapter 23
Kristen M. Swanson
A Program of Research on Caring

Statement of Intent: The intent of this chapter is to offer a rare insight into the personal academic journey of a leading nurse theorist, Kristen Swanson, has chronicled her research on caring and provided an integration of her personal interests with her research activities leading to the development of her caring theory.

Key Terms:

back-and-forth line of inquiry
caring-based therapeutics
knowing
being with
doing for
enabling
maintaining belief
caring
phenomenological analysis
middle-range theory
meta analysis

Chapter Outline:

Turning Point
Predoctoral Experiences
Doctoral Studies
    Dissertation: Caring and Miscarriage
Postdoctoral Study
    Providing Care in the NICU
    Caring for Socially At-Risk Mothers
The Miscarriage Caring Project
    Monitoring Caring as an Intervention Variable
A Literary Meta-analysis of Caring
Summary

Student Objectives/Study Questions:

Following the completion of this chapter students will be able to:

1. Understand back-and-forth line of inquiry.
2. Discuss the evolution of Swanson's research on caring.
3. Understand Swanson's definition of caring and the five caring processes.
4. Explore alternative pathways to developing a research program.
5. Appreciate Swanson's process of development of a program of research.

Transparency Masters (see transparencies 23-1 to 23-3):

23-1 Key to Swanson's Research Program
23-2 Back-and-Forth Line of Inquiry
23-3 Definition of Caring

Chapter 24
Marilyn Anne Ray
The Theory of Bureaucratic Caring

Statement of Intent: The intent of this chapter is to present the theory of bureaucratic caring and its revisioning as holographic theory. The authors offer insight into the process of theory evolution. Practice and education applications of the theory's political and economic dimensions are discussed.

Key Terms:

theory	paradigms
grounded theory	caring
middle-range theory	differential caring
holographic theory	bureaucratic caring
complexity theory	contextual
substantive theory	culture
formal theory	paradox
bureaucracy	informal organization
choice	formal organization

Chapter Outline:

Part 1

Introducing the Theorist

The Theory of Bureaucratic Caring Revisited: From Grounded Theory to
    Holographic Theory

Contemporary Nursing Practice
    The Current Context: Organizational Cultures as Bureaucracies
    Caring as the Unifying Focus of Nursing
    Bureaucratic Caring Theory: Emergent Grounded Theory

Practice Theory Reviewed: Evolution of Theory Development
    Substantive and Formal Theory
    Middle-Range Theory
    Holographic Theory

Revisioning the Theory of Bureaucratic Caring as Holographic Theory
    Reflections on the Theory as Holographic

Summary

Part 2: Applicability of Bureaucratic Caring Theory to Contemporary Nursing Practice: The Political and Economic Dimensions

Current Context of Health-Care Organizations

Review of the Literature: Political and Economic Constraints of Nursing Practice

Economic Implications of Bureaucratic Caring Theory: Research in Current
    Atmosphere of Health-Care Reform
    Challenge to Researchers
    Continued Research on Economics and Caring
    Tool Development

Political/Economic Implication of Bureaucratic Caring
    Health Care and Nursing Administration
    Administrative/Nursing Education
    Nursing Practice

Summary

Student Objectives/Study Questions:

Following the completion of this chapter the student will be able to:

1. Describe what distinguishes organizations as cultures from other paradigms, such as organizations as machines.
2. Identify and discuss characteristics of bureaucracies.
3. Explain the paradox of serving a bureaucracy and serving humans using an example from clinical practice.
4. Identify dimensions of the theory of bureaucratic caring.
5. Compare and contrast the theory of bureaucratic caring and the revised holographic theory of bureaucratic caring.
6. Appreciate the process of theory evolution.

Transparency Masters (see transparencies 24-1 to 24-3):

24-1   Emergence of Theory of Bureaucratic Caring
24-2   Theory of Bureaucratic Caring
24-3   Characteristics of Bureaucracies

Special Sections

Social Section

Sample Course Syllabi

Undergraduate Theory Course (2 credits)

Undergraduate Integrated Course (3 credits)

Graduate Theories and Inquiries Course (3 credits)

College of Nursing
Undergraduate Course Overview

Course Number: NUR 3114

Course Title: Theories of Nursing

Credits: Two Semester Hours

Placement in Curriculum: First Semester Junior Year

Course Description
Theories of nursing are discussed within the context of nursing knowledge, nursing as a discipline and nursing as a professional practice. An overview of nursing theories is presented. The course is designed to prepare students to analyze and evaluate theories of nursing for use in nursing practice.

Course Objectives:
After the completion of the course the student will be able to:
1. Compare and contrast definitions of nursing theory.
2. Describe the usefulness of theory to everyday practice.
3. Discuss the importance of conceptualizing nursing as a discipline of knowledge and professional practice.
4. Articulate enduring personal values and beliefs.
5. Analyze and evaluate extant theories of nursing using a selected guide.
6. Apply selected nursing theories to nursing situations.

Content Outline:
1. Definitions of Nursing
2. Nursing Theory in the Context of Nursing Knowledge
3. Types of Nursing Theory
4. Nursing's Need for Knowledge
5. Reasons for Studying Nursing Theory
6. Choosing a Nursing Theory to Study
7. Analysis and Evaluation of Theory
8. Applying Selected Nursing Theories to Nursing Situations

Teaching Strategies:
Lecture and class discussions
Small-group Work
Assigned Readings
Video Presentations
Written Assignments

Evaluation Methods:

Instructors may choose from the following options:
Midterm Exam
Final Exam
Exercise for the Study of Nursing Theory (see Chapter 2)
Written Assignment on Selected Theorist (using guidelines in Chapter 3)
Group Oral Critique of Nursing Theorist (using guidelines in Chapter 3)
Campaign Election (see Wissmann Annotated Bib. pp)
Theory Building Exercise (see Bevis Annotated Bib. pp)
Reflective Journal of Readings

Required Texts:

Parker, M.E. (2000). *Nursing Theories and Nursing Practice.* Philadelphia: F.A. Davis.

College of Nursing
Integrated Undergraduate Course Overview

Course Number: NUR 3118   3 Credit Hours

Course Title: The Discipline and Profession of Nursing

Placement in Curriculum: Departmental Consent

Course Description: An introduction to nursing as a distinct discipline of knowledge a unique professional practice. Foundational concepts studied include: images of nurse and nursing; nursing as a discipline of knowledge; nursing theories; and nursing as a professional practice.

Course Objectives: On completion of this course the student will:

1. Develop an appreciation of images of nurse and nursing over time held by:
   a. students of nursing
   b. nurses in practice
   c. other health care workers
   d. society

2. Express an understanding of nursing as a discipline of knowledge, including:
   a. characteristics of disciplines of knowledge
   b. ways of knowing fundamentals to nursing
   c. major theoretical conceptions of nursing
   d. conception of nursing held by the College of Nursing faculty
   e. modes of inquiry
   f. relationships among disciplines

3. Express an understanding of nursing as profession, including:
   a. characteristics of a profession and professionhood
   b. social responsibility and accountability
   c. personal and professional leadership
   d. values, standards, ethical and legal systems
   e. education patterns

Content Outline:

1. Images of Nurse and Nursing
   a. Personal Perspectives
   b. Patterns of Knowing
   c. Historical and Philosophical Perspectives
   d. College of Nursing Philosophy

2. Nursing as a Discipline
   a. Characteristics of Disciplines
   b. Theory Development Processes
   c. Major Conceptualizations of Nursing

3. Nursing as a Profession
   a. Characteristics of Professions
   b. Ethical Foundations of Nursing
   c. Internal and External Governance Systems
   d. Social Roles and Patterns of Preparation
   e. Social Contexts

Teaching Strategies:

Lecture
Dialogue
Small-group Discussion
Selected and Assigned Readings
Audiovisuals
Group Presentations

Evaluation Methods:

Instructors may choose from the following options:
Reaction Papers
Midterm Exam
Theory Building Exercise (see Bevis: Annotated Bibliography)
 Final Exam
Campaign Election (see Wissman: Annotated Bibliography)

Required Texts:

Parker, M.E. (2000). *Nursing Theories and Practice.* Philadelphia: F.A. Davis.

Publication Manual of the American Psychological Association (4th ed.). (1994). Washington, D.C.: American Psychological Association.

College of Nursing
Graduate Theory and Inquiry Course
Overview

Course Number: NGR 6201

Course Title: Nursing Theories and Inquiry

Credit Hours: 3 Credits

Placement in Curriculum Core Course in Nursing

Prerequisite: Required course in the first semester of full-time work.

Course Description: This course focuses on the relationships among nursing philosophies, theories and inquiries. Philosophies of science, nursing theories and the foundations for research are analyzed. The goal of the course is to ground inquiry in nursing as a discipline.

Course Objectives: On completion of the course, the student should be able to:

1. Express an understanding of inquiry as an attribute of nursing and the implications of this concept for the development of nursing knowledge and nursing practice.
2. Demonstrate an integrated understanding of the relationships among philosophies of science and nursing theories as they are linked to inquiry.
3. Critique examples of nursing inquiry in reference to their philosophical and theoretical groundings.
4. Formulate researchable questions that have significance for nursing and health care.
5. Perform a review of the literature pertaining to selected topics, and derive conclusions from the review of literature that are related to research questions/hypotheses.

Content Outline:

1. Stance Toward Theory in Nursing
   a. Beliefs About How Knowledge Develops
   b. Beliefs About Human Beings, Environment and Health: Interrelationships Among Metaparadigms
   c. Beliefs About Nursing: Definitions of Nursing and Antecedents to Nursing Situations According to Nurse Theorists
   d. Theorizing in Practice Situations

2. Approaches to Inquiry into the Practice of Nursing
   a. A Priori/a Posteriori Type of Inquiry: Differences and Convergences
   b. The Art of Inquiry in Nursing Practice: Integrating Knowledge from Practice in Light of Theoretical and Empirical Modalities
   c. Skills of Critical Thinking and Inquiry
   d. Paradigms of Inquiry, e.g. Positivist, Postpositivist, Simultaneity
3. Interplay of Inquiry-in-Practice, Empirical and Theoretical Knowledge, Nursing Theories, and Philosophies of Science in the Formulation of Questions for Nursing Research and the Advancement of Nursing Knowledge

Teaching Strategies:
Discussion
Readings
Guided inquiry
Projects
Student Presentations
Inquiry Paper

Evaluation Methods:
Theory Critique Presentation
Clinical Application Paper
Inquiry Paper
Quizzes (2)
Walk Around a Golf Course (see Frank: annotated bibliography)

Required Texts:
Parker, M.E.   (2000).   *Nursing Theories and Practice.* Philadelphia: FA Davis.

Annotated Bibliography of Selected Teaching Strategy Articles

Annotated Bibliography of Selected Teaching Strategy Articles

Creative or novel teaching strategies can be useful when teaching difficult material. The intent of the abstracts in this chapter is to provide selected examples of creative teaching strategies described in the nursing literature. Selected strategies include the use of humor; connecting everyday experiences with theory development; connecting practice situations to understanding theory; role playing; and techniques with uncertain outcomes. Strategies focus on theory development or building, linking theory with nursing practice and linking theory with research.

It is hoped that the selected articles will encourage instructors to have fun and let their imaginations run free in developing innovative approaches to teaching nursing theory.

Where possible, the use of the strategy in undergraduate or graduate-level course work is indicated. The bibliography is not intended to be exhaustive.

Selected Teaching Strategy Articles

Bevis, E.O. (1989). Curriculum Building Nursing: A process (3rd ed., pp. 212–214). New York: National League for Nursing.

Em Bevis provides an example of an exercise designed to introduce theory building. The exercise promotes undergraduate student participation in creating an imaginary theory and developing it through four levels of theory development. In the exercise, students are asked to perceive and name a strange-looking imaginary creature and to label the body parts. Next, students are asked to describe each part and how the parts relate to the whole. Following this description, students are asked to predict how the parts work and to state what would promote or inhibit their predictions. The fourth step of the exercise requires students to design a plan to test their earlier predictions or hypotheses. Students are encouraged to let their imaginations run wild! At the completion of the exercise, students are given a hypothesis statement derived from an extant theory and asked to work backwards through the levels of theory building. More advanced students might be encouraged to formulate their own nursing action hypothesis. The learning activity is presented in a handout form and includes sample student responses.

Byers, M.L. (1990). Teaching advanced pediatric nursing in the framework of Watson's Theory of Caring in Nursing. *Maternal-Child Nursing Journal,* *19*(2), 183–184.

The author presents a description of the use of Watson's theory of caring in nursing to plan and develop master's level pediatric nursing courses. Students are asked to examine the interrelationship between the nurse's caring role and the scientific knowledge needed to carry out the role. The courses are structured around Watson's 10 carative factors with an emphasis on the development of sensitivity to self and others. Outcomes include learning the caring role, experiencing being cared for as a student and enabling the pediatric patient to experience being cared for.

Frank, B. (1994). Teaching nursing theory: A walk around the golf course. *Nurse Educator, 19*(3), 26–27.

Betsy Frank describes a teaching strategy designed to help graduate students see how concrete experiences becomes abstract in the process of theory development. She uses a walk around a university golf course that requires students to observe objects and their relationship to each other. As a group, the class constructs a "theory of golf courses" from their observations. The exercise reinforces the development of theory within the context of prior knowing. A theory of neighborhoods and shopping malls is also addressed. Descriptions of written papers in which students characterize their journey of theory development are presented.

Gordon, N.S. (1998). Influencing mental health nursing practice through the teaching of research and theory: A personal critical review. *Journal of Psychiatric and Mental Health Nursing, 5*(2), 119–1128.

The author reviews factors influencing the teaching of theory and research to mental health nurses. A casework-based curriculum example is provided that emphasizes knowledge and skill development from within the context of clinical experience.

Jacobs-Kramer, M.K. & Huether, S.E. (1988). Curricular considerations for teaching nursing theory. *Journal of Professional Nursing, 4*(5), 373–380.

The authors consider such elements as timing, integration of specific content processes, and content inclusion in the development of undergraduate nursing programs. They believe the quality of rapidly growing doctoral programs of nursing depends on the early introduction of skills related to abstract thought processes. They focus on demystifying theory and emphasize building on everyday theoretical skills. Suggestions for course development including written assignments are provided.

Laschinger, H.K., Docherty, S. D. & Dennis C. (1992). Helping students use nursing models to guide practice. *Nurse Educator, 17*(2), 36–38.

The authors describe a teaching strategy designed to help undergraduate nursing students understand the importance of situating research questions within nursing theoretical frameworks. Working in consultation with graduate teaching assistants (TAs), students were required to develop research questions and place them within nursing conceptual frameworks. Examples of student-generated questions that were transformed to reflect explicit nursing frameworks are provided. Common difficulties are described.

Reed, P. G. (1985). Strategies for teaching nursing research: Theory and metatheory in an undergraduate research course. *Western Journal of Nursing Research, 7*(4), 482–485.

Pamela Reed offers a description of five theory content units developed for an undergraduate research course. The units provide an approach to enable students to raise clinical research questions that are linked to theoretical frameworks.

Smith, B.E. (1992). Linking theory and practice in teaching basic nursing skills. *Journal of Nursing Education, 31*(1), 16–23.

Blenda Smith presents a research study exploring the use of Vee heuristic and concept maps as strategies to identify and reinforce connections between theory and practice in an undergraduate nursing program. Findings support the use of these strategies. A literature review describes the use of these strategies to organize and understand knowledge. Samples of a concept map and Vee heuristic are provided.

Wissmann, J.L. (1994). Teaching nursing theory through an election campaign framework. *Nurse Educator, 19*(5), 21-23.

Jeanne Wissmann presents a teaching-learning strategy requiring students to select and investigate a nursing theorist and apply the theorist's work to nursing practice. The strategy uses the framework of an election campaign. Students are required to manage the "campaign" of a nurse theorist running for vice president of the Nursing Theory Club. Working in small groups, students develop campaign materials, campaign displays and campaign speeches providing an assessment of the individual theorists. Campaign guidelines, rules and evaluation criteria are provided. Written campaign materials were evaluated on the level of analysis of the selected theorist and Sister Callista Roy, who was identified as the theory club president. This fun, participatory strategy was used with BSN completion students.

Guidelines for the Use of Theory in Practice, Administration, and Research

A Guide for Study of Nursing Theory for Use in Practice

1. How is nursing conceptualized in the theory?

   Is the focus of nursing stated?
   > What does the nurse attend to when practicing nursing?
   > What guides nursing observations, reflections, decisions and actions?
   > What does the nurse think about when considering nursing?
   > What are illustrations of use of the theory to guide practice?

   What is the purpose of nursing?
   > What do nurses do when they are practicing nursing?
   > What are exemplars of nursing assessments, designs, plans, evaluations?
   > What indicators give evidence of quality and quantity of nursing practice?
   > Is the richness and complexity of nursing practice evident?

   What are the boundaries or limits for nursing?
   > How is nursing distinguished from other health and medical services?
   > How is nursing related to other disciplines and services?
   > What is the place of nursing in interdisciplinary settings?
   > What is the range of nursing situations in which the theory is useful?

   How can nursing situations be described?
   > What are attributes of the one nursed?
   > What are characteristics of the nurse?
   > How can interactions of the nurse and the one nursed be described?
   > Are there environmental requirements for the practice of nursing?

2. What is the context of development of the theory?

   Who is the nursing theorist as person and as nurse?
   > Why did the theorist develop the theory?
   > What is the background of the theorist as nursing scholar?

   What are the major theoretical influences on this theory?
   > What nursing models and theories influenced this theory?
   > What are the relationships of this theory with other theories?
   > What nursing-related theories and philosophies influenced this theory?

   What were major external influences on development of the theory?
   > What were social, economic, and political influences?
   > What images of nurses and nursing influenced the theory?
   > What was the status of nursing as a discipline and profession?

3. Who are authoritative sources for information about development, evaluation, and use of this theory?

Who are nursing authorities who speak, write about, and use the theory?
What are professional attributes of these persons?
What are attributes of authorities and how does one become one?
Which other nurses should be considered authorities?

What major resources are authoritative sources on the Theory?
Books? Articles? Audio-Visual media? Electronic media?
What nursing societies share and support work of the theory?
What service and academic programs are authoritative sources?

A Guide for Study of Nursing Theory for Use in Administration

1. What are the purposes of the organization?
   Missions?
   Goals?

2. What are the purposes of nursing?
   How do these purposes contribute to the purposes of the organization?

3. How can the range of nursing situations be described?
   What is the population served?

4. What nursing and related technologies are required for nursing?

5. What are the projections for nursing situations and technological need for the future?

6. How is communication facilitated?
   In nursing?
   Among disciplines and services?

7. How are services for those nursed coordinated?

8. In what ways is nursing professional development achieved?
   Career advancement?

9. How are research and development of nursing practice and theory advanced?

A Guide for Study of Nursing Theory for Use in Research

1. How can the overall significance of the theory to nursing research be described?

   What are the phenomena of interest in the theory?

   Can the theory provide plausible explanations of phenomena of interest to nursing?

   What is the scope or range of the theory?

   What is the potential impact of the theory on practice?

2. Is the theory testable?

   Can theory constructs be observed?

   What is the highest level of measurement of the constructs?

   Are explicit propositions measurable?

   Is the theory internally consistent?

   Can meaningful hypothesis statements be formulated?

   Can hypotheses derived from the theory be proved false?

3. What is the experience of nurse researchers who report use of the theory?

   Has the theory been used to guide nursing research?

   What is the explanatory power of the theory?

   What is the predictive power of the theory?

   Has nursing research lead to further theory formulations?

   Has the theory influenced design of nursing research methodology?

   Has the theory been a useful heuristic devise?

   Has the theory been useful in organizing extant knowledge?

Transparencies

Theories Are Not Discovered in Nature.
They Are Invented.

Theories Are Reflections of Human:

- Observations
- Projections
- Inferences

Functions of Theory

- Organize Knowing

- Explain Experience

- Interpret Observation

- Describe Relationships

- Guide Actions

- Predict Outcomes

- Provide Evidence of Achievements

Phenomena of Interest to Nursing

- Focus of Nursing
- Person, Group, or Population Nursed
- Relationship of Nurse and Nursed
- Hoped-for Goals or Purposes of Nursing

Characteristics of Nursing as a Discipline

- Expression of Human Imagination
- Domain
- Syntactical and Conceptual Structures
- Specialized Language and Symbols
- Heritage of Literature
- Communication Networks
- Tradition
- Values and Beliefs
- Education Systems

Characteristics of Nursing as Professional Practice

- Clinical Scholarship
- Processes of Nursing
- Practice Is the Source and Goal of Theory
- Critical Thinking
- Ethical Responsibility
- Evaluate Practice Outcomes
- Theory-Based Research

Sensitizing Questions

- Why Study Nursing Theory?
- What Does the Practicing Nurse Want from Nursing Theory?

Reasons for Studying Nursing Theory

- Everyday Practice Enriches Theory
- Practice and Theory Guided by Values and Beliefs
- Reframe Thinking about Nursing
- Theory Guides Use of Ideas and Techniques
- Close Gap Between Theory and Research
- Envision Potentialities

Central Belief

The study and use of nursing theory in nursing practice must have roots in the everyday practice of nurses.

Issues Important to the Study of Nursing Theory

- Personal Nursing Practice
- Personal Interests, Abilities, and Experiences
- Resources and Support
- Theorist, Evidence, and Opinion

Steps in Choosing a Nursing Theory to Guide Practice

- Reflection on Values and Beliefs
- Identification of Major Components of Nursing Situations
- Connecting Values and Nursing Situations
- Verifying Awareness and Appreciation
- Choosing a Theory for Study
- Using Authoritative Sources
- Choosing a Theory Analysis and Evaluation Guide

Study of Nursing Theory for Use in Practice Guide

- Conceptualization of Nursing
- Context of Theory Development
- Authoritative Sources
- Overall Significance

Study of Nursing Theory for Use in Nursing Administration Guide

- Purposes of the Organization
- Purposes of Nursing
- Range of Nursing Situations
- Nursing and Related Technologies
- Projections of Needs
- Communication Facilitation
- Professional Nursing Development
- Practice Research and Development

Health of Houses

- Ventilation
- Light
- Cleanliness
- Taking of food
- Interpersonal milieu

Major Factors Influencing Nightingale's Model

- Religion
- Science
- War
- Feminism

Nightingale's Assumptions

1. Nursing is separate from medicine.

2. Nurses should be trained.

3. Environment is important to health.

4. Disease process is not important to nursing.

5. Nursing should support environment.

6. Research is utilized through observation and empirics.

7. Nursing is both science and art.

8. Nursing's concern is the person in the environment.

9. Person interacts with environment.

10. Sick and well are governed by laws of health.

11. Nurse should be observant and confidential.

Hildegard E. Peplau

Born September 1, 1909 in Reading, Pennsylvania

1931: Graduated; Pottstown, Pennsylvania, Hospital School of Nursing

College: Head Nurse and Executive Officer of Health Service at Bennington College, Vermont

Bachelor's degree in Interpersonal Psychology

1948: Master's in Psychiatric Mental Health Nursing from Columbia University

1952: Interpersonal Relations in Nursing

Framework for the practice of psychiatric nursing

1955: Began her Clinical Nurse Specialist at Rutgers where she remained until 1974 when she retired

1994: American Academy of Nursing Living Legends Hall of Fame

11 Honorary Degrees

1998: American Nurses Association Hall of Fame

Mentor of many

3-Step Process of Practice-Based Theory Development
by
Hildegard E. Peplau

1. Observations are made in practice: name, categorize, and classify the phenomenon.

   a. participant observation
   b. spectator observation
   c. interviewer and random observation

2. Decode and categorize data and identify layers of meaning at different levels of abstraction in order to apply a conceptual framework to a particular phenomenon.

3. Useful interventions are derived and tested.

"Interventions . . . assisted patients in gaining interpersonal and intellectual competencies evolved through the nurse-patient relationship" Otoole & Welt, 1989, p. 351.

(Peplau, 1989)
Induction to Deduction

Peplau . . . always ahead of her time provided an approach to knowledge development through the scholarship of practice: nursing knowledge is developed in practice as well as for practice (Reed, 1996, p. 29).

Peplau . . . used clinical situations to inductively derive theories that were tested in clinical practice. She also applied existing social theory to nursing phenomena.

The process of combining induction (observation and classification) with deduction (application of known concepts to data) provides a creative, nonlinear approach to the formation of ideas.

This methodology naturally links qualitative and quantitative methods of research to practice.

Essence of a Philosophy

- Reverence for the Gift of Life
- Respect for Human Beings
  —dignity
  —autonomy
  —worth
  —individuality
- Resolution to Act Dynamically in Relation to Beliefs

Prescriptions Specify

- Nature of Action
- Determining Thinking Process

Kinds of Deliberate Action

- Mutually Understood and Agreed Upon
- Patient Directed
- Nurse Directed

Essential Ingredients of Prescriptive Theory

- The Nurse's Central Purpose in Nursing
- The Prescription
- The Realities

Features of Practice Realities

- Nurse as Agent
- Patient as Recipient
- Recognition of Framework by Nurse and Patient
- Goal of Nursing
- Awareness of Means

Steps in Reaching Goals

- Goal in Intent
  —specifies patient attitude
- Goal in Application
  —specifies nursing framework
- Goal in Execution
  —specifies relationship between realities and activity

Theory and Clinical Practice

"The practice of clinical nursing is goal directed, deliberately carried out, and patient centered" (Wiedenbach, 1964, p. 23).

Paradigmatic Origins

- Nightingale
- Systems Theory
- Developmental Theory

Five Core Principles

- Wholeness and Order
- Stabilization
- Reorganization
- Hierarchic Interaction
- Dialectical Contradiction

Subsystems

- Achievement
- Affiliative
- Aggressive/Protective
- Dependency
- Eliminative
- Ingestive
- Restorative
- Sexual

Definitions

- Person: Behavioral system
- Environment: Internal and external
- Health: Functioning of the system
- Nursing and Nursing Therapeutics: Contribution to the health and well-being of people

Myra Levine's Conservation Model Assumptions

1. All nursing actions are moral actions.

2. Human beings respond in a singular yet integrated fashion.

3. Each individual responds wholly and completely to every alteration in his life pattern.

4. Individuals cannot be understood out of the context of their environment.

5. "Ultimately decisions for nursing care are based on the unique behavior of the individual patient . . ." (Levine, 1973, p. 6).

6. "Patient centered care means individualized nursing care . . ." (Levine, 1973, p. 23).

7. "Every self sustaining system monitors its own behavior by conserving the use of resources required to define its unique identity" (Levine, 1973, p. 4).

8. The nurse is responsible for recognizing the state of altered health and the patient's organismic response to altered health.

9. Nursing is a unique contributor to patient care.

10. The patient is in an altered state of health.

11. Guardian Angel assumes that the nurse accepts responsibility and shows concern based on knowledge that makes it possible to decide in the patient's behalf.

Levine's Conservation Model Values

1. All nursing actions are moral actions.

2. Two moral imperatives are the sanctity of life and the relief of suffering.

3. Ethical behavior "is the day to day expression of one's commitment to other persons and the ways in which human beings relate to one another in their daily interactions" (Levine, 1977, p. 846).

4. A fully informed individual should make decisions regarding life and death in advance of the situations. These decisions are not the role of the health care provider or family (Levine, 1989).

5. Judgements by nurses or doctors about quality of life are inappropriate and should not be used as a basis for the allocation of care (Levine, 1989b).

6. "Persons who require the intensive interventions of critical care units enter with a contract of trust. To respect trust . . . is a moral responsibility" (Levine, 1988b, p. 88).

Levine's Conservation Model Organismic Responses

1. **Response to fear (fight/flight response).**
   Most primitive: instantaneous; real or perceived threats.

2. **Inflammatory response.**
   Second level: structural integrity and promotion of healing.

3. **Response to stress.**
   Third level: prolonged exposure to stressful experience.

4. **Perceptual response.**
   Fourth level: gathering environment information and converting it to meaning.

Ida Jean Orlando, August 12, 1926 The Dynamic Nurse–Patient Relationship

Nursing is responsive to individuals who suffer or anticipate a sense of helplessness; it is focused on the process of care in an immediate experience; it is concerned with providing direct assistance to individuals in whatever setting they are found for the purpose of avoiding, relieving, diminishing, or curing the individual's sense of helplessness (Orlando, 1972).

Dynamic Nurse–Patient Relationship Ida Jean Orlando

GOAL: Interpersonal process aimed at assisting patients when they are experiencing distress.

Nursing—deliberative interaction process that is learned and includes patient needs, nurse's reaction, and nursing interventions
Nursing practice—interaction process focused on patient needs and response to the environment

FIT: Inductive theory based on the study of clinical practice. Emphasis on nurse–patient relationship as the vehicle for achieving the goals.

UNDERSTANDABILITY: Common wording contributes to the easy usage of this theory.

CONTROL: General theory for nursing interactions and interpersonal relationships with patients and is not focused on particular populations, so control is weak in specific situations.

Aspects of Person as Patient

- Person
- Body
- Disease

Loeb Center RNs

- Chief Therapeutic Agents
- Provide All Hands-on Care
- Responsible for Total Health Program

Deterrents to Replicating Loeb Center Model

- Different Definition of Professional Nursing
- Value Conflicts
- Economic Incentives
- Concerns over Patient Census
- Challenges to Existing Power

People Influencing Henderson's Search for a Personal Definition of Nursing

Caroline Stackpole: *Principle of Physiological Balance*

Edward Thorndike: *Fundamental Needs of Man Framework*

Dr. George Deaver: *Individualized Programs of Care and Constant Evaluation*

Questions Directing Henderson's Search for a Definition of Nursing

"What is Nursing that is not also medicine, physical therapy, social work, etc.?"

"What is the unique function of the nurse?"

(Henderson & Harmer, 1955, p. 4)

Henderson's Definition of Nursing

"Nursing is primarily assisting the individual (sick or well) in the performance of those activities contributing to health or its recovery, (or to a peaceful death), that he would perform unaided if he had the necessary strength, will, or knowledge. It is likewise the unique contribution of nursing to help people be independent of such assistance as soon as possible."

(Harmer & Henderson, 1955, p. 4)

Henderson's Basic Nursing Care Components

1. Breathe normally.

2. Eat and drink adequately.

3. Eliminate body wastes.

4. Move and maintain desirable postures.

5. Sleep and rest.

6. Select suitable clothes—dress and undress.

7. Maintain body temperature within normal range by adjusting clothing and modifying the environment.

8. Keep the body clean and well groomed and protect the integument.

Henderson's Basic Nursing Care Components (Continued)

9. Avoid dangers in the environment and avoid injuring others.

10. Communicate with others in expressing emotions, needs, fears, or opinions.

11. Worship according to one's faith.

12. Work in such a way that there is a sense of accomplishment.

13. Play or participate in various forms of recreation.

14. Learn, discover, or satisfy the curiosity that leads to normal development and health, and use the available health facilities.

Basic Nursing Care Components

- Reflect:

  Personal hygiene needs

  Healthful living needs

- Outline:

  Functions nurses control and initiate

  Boundaries for nursing practice

Questions Henderson Used to Evaluate Nursing Care

- What did I do to help you?
- What did I do that didn't help you?
- What did I not think of that might have helped you?

(Birnbach, 1998, p. 45)

Statement on Independent Practice

"It is my contention that the nurse is, and should legally be, an independent practitioner and able to make independent judgments as long as he or she is not diagnosing, prescribing treatment for disease, or making a prognosis, for these are the physician's functions."

(Henderson, 1966, *The Nature of Nursing*, p. 22)

World of Others and Things

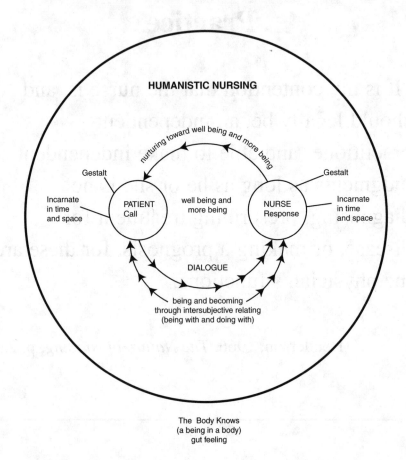

HUMANISTIC NURSING

nurturing toward well being and more being

Gestalt

Gestalt

Incarnate
in time
and space

PATIENT
Call

well being and
more being

NURSE
Response

Incarnate
in time
and space

DIALOGUE

being and becoming
through intersubjective relating
(being with and doing with)

The Body Knows
(a being in a body)
gut feeling

Shared Human Experience

Nursing is Transactional

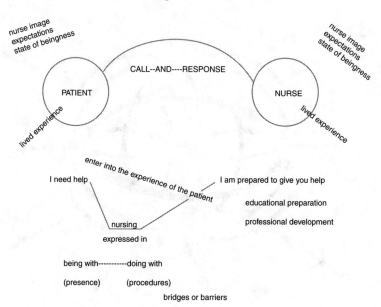

Patient and Nurse Gestalts "Between"

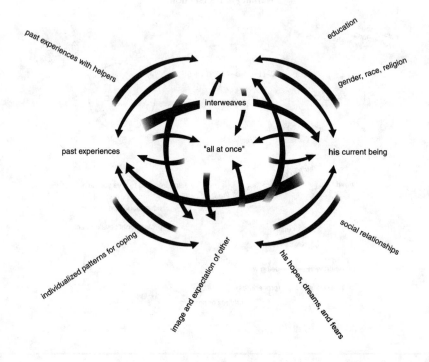

Phases of Humanistic Nursing Inquiry

- Preparation of the Nurse Knower

- Nurse Knowing the Other Intuitively

- Nurse Knowing the Other Scientifically

- Nurse Complementarily Synthesizing Known Others

- Succession Within the Nurse from the Many to the Paradoxical One

Nurse Complimentarily Synthesizing Others

Dialectic

a new overall grasp

sudden insights

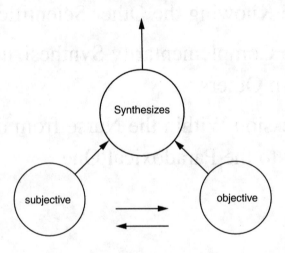

Noetic Loci

"knowing place"

Eleven Phenomena of Nursing

- Awareness
- Openness
- Empathy
- Caring
- Touching
- Understanding
- Responsibility
- Trust
- Acceptance
- Self-Recognition
- Dialogue

Sensitizing Question

What is nursing's phenomenon of concern?

Role of Nursing

Nursing enables individuals to develop and exercise their self-care abilities to the extent that they can provide for themselves the amount and quality of care required.

Self-Care Deficit Theory of Nursing Concepts

- Self-Care
- Self-Care Agency
- Therapeutic Self-Care Demand
- Self-Care Deficit
- Nursing Agency
- Nursing Systems

Historical Perspective of Martha Elizabeth Rogers

Born: May 12, 1914—same day as Florence Nightingale

Knoxville General Hospital Nursing Program

George Peabody College of Nashville Tennessee

Bachelor's degree in Public Health Nursing

Teacher's College, Columbia University

Master's degree in Nursing

Johns Hopkins University in Baltimore, Maryland

Master's degree in public health

Doctor of Science

1954 became Head of Division of Nursing at
New York University

Wrote *Educational Revolution in Nursing*, 1961

Reveille in Nursing 1964: *An Introduction to the
Theoretical Basis of Nursing*, 1970

Helped draft and get passed the Nurse Practice Act

Founded Society for Advancement in Nursing in 1974

Died 1994

(*Martha E. Rogers, Her Life and Her Work* edited by
Malinski and Barrett, 1994)

Rogers' Unique View of Nursing

NURSING IS A SCIENCE!

"Irreducible human being and its environment, both identified as energy fields"

"Pandimensional view of people and their world"

"Nonlinear domain without spatial or temporal attributes"

We are already living in a new reality, one that is "a synthesis of rapidly evolving, accelerating ways of using knowledge" (Rogers, 1994a, p. 33).

Rogers' Principles of Homeodynamics

- Resonancy
- Helicy
- Integrality

Rogerian Practice Model

- Barrett's Rogerian Practice Methodology for Health Patterning
  —Pattern manifestation appraisal
  —Deliberative mutual patterning

- Cowling's Pattern Appreciation Practice Method " being thankful or grateful for; enjoying or understanding critically or emotionally" (Cowling, 1997, p. 130).
  —Pattern manifestation knowing and appreciation

- Voluntary Mutual Patterning

Discipline of Nursing Paradigmatic Perspectives Parse Theory

Totality paradigm: Human as body-mind-spirit—particulate focusing on whole human as they interact with and adapt to the environment.

Simultaneity paradigm: Human as unitary—irreducible in mutual process with the universe.

Man-Living-Health: A theory of nursing
Parse, 1981

changed to

The Human Becoming School of Thought
Parse, 1998

Now includes three research methodologies
and a unique practice methodology

Making it a School of Thought
Not Just a Theory

Assumptions of Human Becoming from Parse Model

Nine fundamental assumptions:
Four assumptions concerning "Humans"
Five assumptions concerning "Becoming"

From these nine assumptions arise three major themes:

- Meaning
  —Imaging
  —Valuing
  —Languaging

- Rhythmicity
  —Revealing-concealing
  —Enabling-limiting
  —Connecting-separating

- Transcendence
  —Powering
  —Originating
  —Transforming

Research Methodologies from Parse Model

Two Basic Research Methods:*

1. Parse Method—uses participants' descriptions

2. Hermeneutic method—uses written texts and art forms

*The purpose of these two methods is to advance the science of human becoming by studying lived experiences.

Applied Research Method*

1. Descriptive qualitative preproject-process-postproject method

*Popular, often used method that evaluates the changes, satisfactions and effectiveness of health care.

Stages of Binding and Unbinding

1. Potential Freedom

2. Binding

3. Centering

4. Choice

5. Decentering

6. Unbinding

7. Real Freedom

Caring in the Human Health Experience

- Particulate-deterministic
- Interactive-integrative
- Unitary-transformative

HEC Research Process

The Interview

Transcription

The Narrative

Diagram

Follow-up

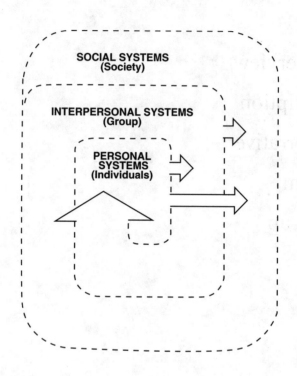

Definition of System

Series of functional components connected by communication links exhibiting purposeful goal-directed behavior. (King, 1996)

Process of Concept Development and Validation

- Review, Analyze, and Synthesize Research Literature
- Identify Concept Attributes
- Write a Conceptual Definition
- Select/Develop Instrument
- Design a Study
- Select a Population
- Collect Data
- Analyze and Interpret Data
- Write Findings & Conclusions
- Nursing Knowledge Implications

Sensitizing Question

What is the nature of human beings?

Goal of Nursing

Help individuals maintain or regain health.
(King, 1990)

Adaptive Modes

- Physiologic–Physical

- Self-Concept–Group Identity

- Role Function

- Interdependence

Central Belief of the Roy Adaptation Model

Adaptive Responses Support Health

Topics for Research

- Cognator–Regulator Effectiveness

- Stabilizor–Innovator Effectiveness

- Adaptive Modes

- Nursing Care Promoting Adaptive
  Processes

Knowledge Development Strategies Based On The Roy Adaptation Model

- Model Construction

- Theory Development
  —concept analysis
  —derivation of propositional statements
  —philosophic explication

- Instrument Development

Betty Neuman's Systems Model

- Primary Prevention: general knowledge that is applied in an effort to promote client wellness by stressor prevention and reduction of risk factors

- Secondary prevention: relates to reaction to stressors, appropriate ranking of intervention priorities, and treatment to reduce their noxious effects

- Tertiary prevention: adjustive processes taking place, a reconstitution begins, and maintenance factors move the client back in a circular manner toward primary prevention

Neuman's Five Client Variables

- Physiological: bodily structure and function
- Psychological: mental processes and relationships
- Sociocultural: combined social and cultural functions
- Developmental: life developmental processes
- Spiritual: spiritual belief influence (Neuman, 1995b, p. 28)

Role of Nurse

Neuman (1995b) believes the nurse creates a linkage among the client, the environment, health and nursing in the process of keeping the system stable.

Major Conceptual Elements

- Carative Factors (clinical Caritas Processes)
- Transpersonal Caring Relationship
- Caring Moment/Caring Occasion
- Caring (Healing) Consciousness

Original Carative Factors

1. Formation of a humanistic-altruistic system of values

2. Instillation of faith-hope

3. Cultivation of sensitivity to one's self and to others

4. Development of a helping trusting, human caring relationship

5. Promotion and acceptance of the expression of positive and negative feelings

Original Carative Factors (Continued)

6. Systematic use of a creative problem-solving caring process

7. Promotion of transpersonal teaching-learning

8. Provision for a supportive, protective, and/or corrective mental, physical, societal, and spiritual environment

9. Assistance with gratification of human needs

10. Allowance for existential-phenomenological-spiritual forces

Role of Consciousness
Consciousness is:

- Contained
- Interconnected
- Communicated to the one being cared for
- Exists through and transcends time and space

(Watson, 1992, p. 148)

Effective Caring Leader Questions

1. What is the nature of the human being and what does he/she need to experience fulfillment?

2. What is the basis for harmonious and productive human relationships?

3. What is the nature of health/healing?

4. What is the purpose/mission of the organization or work team?

Rationale for Transcultural Nursing

- Global migration
- Cultural problems and cultural conflicts
- Consumer fears and resistance to health personnel
- Different cultures frustrated and misunderstood by health personnel
- Health personnel frustrated/angry when clients fail to cooperate
- Consumers of different cultures dissatisfied with care
- Intercultural conflicts in health care settings
- Nurses lack of cultural knowledge

Transcultural Nursing

"Formal area of study (education and research) and practice focused on the cultural care (caring) values, beliefs, and practices of individuals or groups from a particular culture in order to provide culture-specific care to people of diverse cultures." (Leininger, 1995)

Culturally Congruent Care Modalities

- Preservation or Maintenance
- Accommodation or Negotiation
- Restructuring or Repatterning of Care

Purpose of Culture Care Theory

- Discover
- Document
- Analyze
- Interpret

Goal of Culture Care Theory

To provide research-based knowledge in order to provide culturally congruent, safe, and beneficial care to people of diverse and similar cultures.

Assumptions

1. Persons are caring by virtue of their humanness.

2. Persons are whole and complete in the moment.

3. Persons live caring moment to moment.

4. Personhood is a way of living grounded in caring.

5. Personhood is enhanced through participation in nurturing relationships with caring others.

6. Nursing is both a discipline and a profession.

Caring

"Caring is the intentional and authentic presence of the nurse with another who is recognized as living caring and growing in caring."

Key Themes

- Focus and Intention of Nursing
- Nursing Situation
- Personhood
- Call for Nursing
- "Caring Between"
- Lived Meaning of Nursing as Caring

Coming to Know Self

- Trusting in Self
- Learning to Let Go
- Being Open and Humble
- Continuous Calling to Consciousness
- Taking Time to Fully Experience
- Finding Hope in the Moment

Frequently Asked Questions

1. How do nurses come to know self and others?

2. Must I like my patients to serve them?

3. What about nursing a person for whom it is difficult to care?

4. Is it possible to nurse someone who is in an unconscious or altered state of awareness?

5. How does nursing process fit with this theory?

6. How practical is this theory in the real world of nursing?

Key to Swanson's Research Program

The study of human responses to a specific health problem (miscarriage) in a framework (caring) that assumed a clinical therapeutic be defined.

Back-and-Forth Line of Inquiry

- What's wrong? What can be done?
- What's right? How can it be strengthened?
- What's real to individuals experiencing a specific health problem?

Swanson's Definition of Caring

"A nurturing way of relating to a valued other toward whom one feels a personal sense of commitment."

Theory of Bureaucratic Caring Emerged from the Worldviews of Health Professionals and Patients in Practice.

Theory of Bureaucratic Caring Can Be Viewed as

- Grounded Theory
- Middle-range theory
- Grand theory

Characteristics of Bureaucracies

- Fixed Division of Labor
- Hierarchy of Offices
- Set of General Rules
- Separation of Personnel from Officials
- Selection Based on Technical Qualifications
- Standards of Fairness—Equal Treatment
- Employment Viewed as Career
- Dismissal Protection by Tenure